SPEAKING RACE IN HEALTHCARE

A Manual for a New Dialogue

MILAGROS PHILLIPS

SPEAKING RACE IN HEALTHCARE

A Manual for a New Dialogue

Cover Design by Milagros Phillips

© 2018 by Milagros Phillips

All rights reserved

ISBN-10: 1729642985

ISBN-13: 978-1729642986

DEDICATION

This book is dedicated to the countless men and women who want to speak about the effects of racism on the health of their organizations, clients, and patients with their colleagues, clients, and patients and don't quite know how to facilitate those conversations. It is also dedicated to people of color who suffer higher incidents of diseases.

A Manual for a New Dialogue

CONTENTS

FOREWORD 1

INTRODUCTION 5

GLOSSARY OF TERMS 9

RACE & HEALTH OUTCOMES 13

    WHY RACE IN THE HEALTH CONVERSATION 14

WHAT IS RACE LITERACY? 19

INTERGENERATIONAL AND HISTORICAL TRAUMA 23

SELF-PREPARATION 29

    CLARITY IS KEY 33

    CONFRONTATION 33

    ALLOW THE PROCESS 34

    MAKE ROOM FOR THE UNEXPECTED 36

    PREPARE FOR CRITICISM 37

THE SETUP 39

    WHERE IS THE CONVERSATION TAKING PLACE? ... 40

    THE PURPOSE 40

    BE CLEAR ABOUT THE PURPOSE OF THE
        CONVERSATION 42

    FOLLOW-UP 42

RULES OF ENGAGEMENT 45

A Manual for a New Dialogue

- THE RULES FOR SHARING 47
- QUESTIONS TO CONSIDER 49
- CREATING A SAFE SPACE 49
- PERSONAL HISTORY WITH RACE 50
- ENCOUNTERING DIFFERENCES........................... 51
- PREPARE FOR OVERTIME 53

HISTORY 55

EXPERIENCE 61

RACE IN THE HEALTHCARE ORGANIZATION 75

- WHAT IS AFFECTED IN THE ORGANIZATION? 78

THE CONVERSATION 81

- COMPONENTS OF THE CONVERSATION ....
- TELLING 81

LISTENING AND HEARING 85

- QUESTIONS TO CONSIDER 88

QUESTIONING 89

- Hijacking 90
- Resistance 90

EMOTIONS 93

FEELINGS INVENTORY 97

- FEELINGS WHEN NEEDS ARE SATISFIED................ 97
- FEELINGS WHEN NEEDS ARE NOT SATISFIED 99
- QUESTIONS TO CONSIDER 102

THE HEALING CRISIS **105**

WHEN IT SEEMS ENDLESS **109**

CREATING A VISION **113**

    QUESTIONS TO CONSIDER **114**

TAKING ACTION **115**

CONCLUSION **123**

REFERENCES **129**

A Manual for a New Dialogue

ACKNOWLEDGMENTS

With great gratitude, I acknowledge my family and precious friends for their loving support of my ideas of how to leave this world a better place. A special thank you to my Editor, Alexander R. Cohen. I graciously acknowledge Michael L. Robinson and, Supervisor Julie Fitch for their contributions, Meenal Kelkar, Deirdre McGlynn, Fatma Ghedira, and Charles Herald for their help with the technology.

A Manual for a New Dialogue

FOREWORD

Caring for our health is one of the most important things that we can do. Healthcare and Community-based organizations working in underserved communities, often with limited resources and small staffs have a monumental task and do a tremendous job in caring for the health of the community. While these organizations do much-needed work in communities of color, race is a conversation they often avoid.

The medical system and community-based organizations often experience racial miscommunication, fail to identify their problems with race, overlook how race affects the people they serve, and rarely if ever consider the effects of race in creating a treatment plan. In their desire to serve the community, they often leave those they are serving out of the conversation. Conversations on race are mostly avoided, even though communities of color, and in particular African-American communities, suffer the highest numbers when it comes to high blood pressure, diabetes, new HIV cases, infant mortality, and cancer deaths. African-Americans are 50 percent more likely to get lung cancer (despite lower tobacco exposure). Although the people of color fare worse in health numbers, race, racism, the effects of intergenerational, historical trauma, and current trauma, everyday macro and microaggressions faced by people of color, and the burden of excess stress caused by living under a racial caste system are rarely if ever considered as part of the healthcare conversation or addressed as part of treatment.

This manual was created to support organizations that want to have conversations on race with their employees and with the communities that they serve.

Even if an organization has never tackled a conversation on race, it will be able to use this manual. Facilitators will be able to use the manual to get conversations going in their organizations. It is my hope that the those using this handbook will find it a helpful tool to which they can return for guidance on how to speak race in healthcare, over and over again. I also hope that patients and those being served by community-based organizations will find this information helpful in speaking with their healthcare providers. There are many stress reduction techniques that your healthcare providers may recommend, and there are insurance companies that cover these services for their clients. When you have information, it is easier to ask the right questions. Speaking Race in Healthcare and becoming race literate may help you care for yourself, organization, and community in a more informed and expansive way.

A Manual for a New Dialogue

INTRODUCTION

As America struggles with the healthcare crisis, communities of color, in particular, African-American and Latino communities are the most affected. Health disparities, racial biases, and race illiteracy, as well as racial inequity, emphasize the need for a dialogue on race and health, which leads to inspired action.

While the need to speak about race is essential to healthcare, race remains America's taboo. If we are to adhere to culturally and linguistically appropriate services, as outlined by the Department of Health and Human Services, all healthcare providers need to consider race an important part of the healthcare dialogue. Cultural and Linguistically Appropriate Services (CLAS) was established to "advance health equity, improve quality of care, and help eliminate health disparities by establishing a blueprint for health and healthcare organizations." Its guiding principle is that healthcare organizations should "provide effective, equitable, understandable, and respectful quality care and services that are responsive to diverse cultural health beliefs and practices, preferred languages, health literacy, and other communication needs."

Without an understanding of the impact of race on the health of all Americans, both positive and negative, it is difficult to have the often-dreaded conversation. Through no fault of their own, providers often lack the racial literacy to connect the dots, as the history of race in America is not taught in school. Ignorance of their racial biases can get in the way and often affects the way patients/clients are treated. Prejudice and discrimination can block communication. Moreover, when race is broached in a conversation on health, providers often get nervous; concerns about being seen as racist become more important than the patient's/client's well-being. When we make race part of the healthcare conversation on a regular basis, the conversation can be more productive at stressful times.

This book is divided into two parts. Part one is the text, which includes a Glossary of Terms explaining how specific words are used in this book. This part of the book covers a few reasons why the conversation is important and needed. At the end there is a conclusion that includes recommendations for organizations desiring to learn more. Part two is the manual for facilitators. This manual is for anyone wishing to lead a group conversation on race, and the principles are also useful for one-on-one conversations. Whether it is at the dinner table or the boardroom Speaking Race in Healthcare is *the manual for the dialogue.* This manual is available for free at **www.MilagrosPhillips.com**. Just enter you name and email address to receive the free manual.

A Manual for a New Dialogue

GLOSSARY OF TERMS

When it comes to race, there are a lot of terms that are used interchangeably or have different meanings for different people. This glossary is placed here for clarification of these terms as they are used in this book. All sources are referenced in the back of this book. In the cases where I was not able to find a definition or clarification, I created a definition for the purposes of the book.

RACE – A human construct that has been in place since the early 1500s. The creation of human subspecies through classification systems was a way to justify unequal treatment of Africans in bondage for a free labor force. While we no longer adhere to the belief in human subspecies, the unequal treatment persists till today, and it has been institutionalized in our healthcare system.

Racism – Racial prejudice plus power. *"From its inception, prejudice in the hands of those with power has systematically been used to control access to power, education, finances, housing, and even healthcare. By establishing racism as law, one could systematically leave the marginalized populations out of basic human rights and use the law to justify it."* http://www.bluffton.edu/facstaff/damascus/index.html - Bluffton has since taken this link down. However, prejudice plus power is the definition used by anti-racists, and it is the definition used in this book.

RACIST — *"A person who shows or feels discrimination or prejudice against people of other races, or who believes that a particular race is superior to another."* In this manual, the meaning is expanded to include policies, institutions, and practices that are racist.

RACE LITERACY — *"The knowledge and awareness of the history of race, how one is acculturated into a racial caste, the systems in the nation-state that support race as a human divide, and the impact of all of the above on our current events and individual lives."*

PREJUDICE — *"Preconceived opinion that is not based on reason or experience: 'English prejudice against foreigners.' Dislike, hostility, or unjust behavior deriving from preconceived and unfounded opinions: 'accusations of racial prejudice."*

BIAS — *"Inclination or prejudice for or against one person or group, especially in a way considered to be unfair: 'there was evidence of bias against black applicants."*

IMPLICIT BIAS — *"Also known as implicit social cognition, implicit bias refers to the attitudes or stereotypes that affect our understanding, actions, and decisions in an unconscious manner. ... Rather, implicit biases are not accessible through introspection."*

EXPLICIT BIAS — *"Explicit bias refers to the attitudes and beliefs we have about a person or group on a conscious level."*

DISCRIMINATION — *"The unjust or prejudicial treatment of different categories of people, especially on the grounds of race, age, or sex: 'victims of racial discrimination."*

TRAUMA — *"An event or series of events, an experience or prolonged experiences, and/or a threat or perceived threats to a person's well-being."*

SECONDARY TRAUMA — Trauma that affects those witnessing, reading or hearing about another person's the trauma.

TRAUMA-INFORMED CARE — *"A framework of thinking and interventions that are directed by a thorough understanding of the profound neurological, biological, psychological, and social effects trauma has on an individual — recognizing that person's constant interdependent needs for safety, connections, and ways to manage emotions/impulses."*

WHITE PRIVILEGE — *"White privilege (or white skin privilege) is a term for societal privileges that benefit people identified as white in Western countries, beyond what is commonly experienced by non-white (people of color), under the same social, political, or economic circumstances."*

WHOLE PERSON APPROACH – The whole person approach or whole-being approach to healing takes into consideration the individual's mind, body, spirit, and emotions in creating a treatment plan

CHAPTER 1

RACE & HEALTH OUTCOMES

In 1999 Congress requested an Institute of Medicine study to assess the extent of disparities in the types and quality of health services received by U.S. racial and ethnic minorities and non-minorities, explore factors that may contribute to inequities in care, and recommend policies and practices to eliminate these inequities.

The resulting 2002 institute report on unequal treatment concluded, "racial and ethnic disparities in healthcare exist and, because they are associated with worse outcomes in many cases, are unacceptable."

The IOM report defined disparities in healthcare as *"racial or ethnic differences in the quality of healthcare that are not due to access-related factors or clinical needs, preferences, and appropriateness of intervention."*

WHY RACE IN THE HEALTH CONVERSATION

African-Americans bear the greatest burden of diseases such as high blood pressure, diabetes, kidney disease, asthma, lung scarring, and lung cancer. According to WebMD -

- *"Diabetes is 60% more common in black Americans than in white Americans. Blacks are up to 2.5 times more likely to suffer a limb amputation and up to 5.6 times more likely to suffer kidney disease than other people with diabetes.*

- *Despite lower tobacco exposure, black men are 50% more likely than white men to get lung cancer.*
- *Cancer treatment is equally successful for all races. Yet black men have a 40% higher cancer death rate than white men. African-American women have a 20% higher cancer death rate than white women."*

Being able to speak fluently about race is essential to the health of the African-American community. Health practitioners and service providers need to become race literate, understand the effects of intergenerational historical trauma in communities of color, and move past the fear of speaking about race if they are to be part of the solution. Moreover, there are organizational issues that need to be addressed and discussed when it comes to race. Michael L. Robinson, who has worked with community-based organizations since 1997, says:

"Racism within Community Based Organizations (CBO) can be found in many and varied ways, but it is often

very covert in much of the way it is throughout other facets of everyday life today. Racism can permeate an entire CBO, however, is not immediately apparent. When you begin to pull back the layers, you find that it can be so passive aggressive and nuanced that those who suffer from the discourse it produces, might question whether it's really happening to them. They question if they will seem like a trouble-maker if they question what is happening. It can be disguised by strategies such as tokenism, and further covered up by degrees of political correctness. An example is when the organization is asked why there are so few or no People Of Color (POC) in administrative or leadership positions at a particular CBO. The response is, 'We didn't have any qualified (POC) apply for the position."

Michael adds, *"Many CBOs are set up to help the most vulnerable and needy of our communities. Therefore, it is disconcerting when employees at a particular CBOs don't reflect or look like the people they serve. This is a clear indication that the agency does not value the cultural relevance and input of its constituency. This is often the case when some CBOs primarily serve the black community. In response, the CBO may employ the one centralized and publicly visible black person so that the agency has the appearance of caring about the community in which it serves."*

With race affecting the organization and the people that it serves, conversations on race need to be at the forefront of the healthcare agenda on a regular basis. But more than just a willingness to speak about race is needed. Race literacy is required to be able to speak about race and its impact on the lives of the people inside and outside of the organization. Once acknowledged, action needs to be taken to ensure that the causes of the racial disparities are properly addressed.

A Manual for a New Dialogue

CHAPTER 2
WHAT IS RACE LITERACY?

"Race literacy is the knowledge and awareness of the history of race, how one is acculturated into a racial caste, the systems in the nation-state that support race as a human divide, and the impact of all of the above on our current events and individual lives." 11 Reasons to Become Race Literate.

Race literacy helps us understand the intergenerational and historical trauma that is often ignored in healthcare conversations. While practitioners gather health history, this obvious piece of the equation is largely overlooked. The languages that people speak and the amount of melanin in their skin may inform how they are treated and how much information their healthcare provider gives them. It determines whether they will be told what treatment options and medical modalities are available to them. It affects how a patient/client will be spoken to and how much time a practitioner will spend with them.

Race Literacy

- informs our understanding of the current state of race in America
- gives us a broader spectrum of what we mean when we say Race
- gives us a different view of our healthcare system
- creates an opportunity to come up with new solutions

While conversations on race are not easy for many, they are essential to the health of Americans of color and crucial to the health of African-Americans. Conversations on race require quiet listening, time, and energy. They also require care — care for self and care for others who are part of the interchange. Conversations are an exchange of ideas and a sharing of experiences and information that, when done well, leave us better off than we were when we started. Conversations on race as part of the healthcare continuum can save lives. Whether the conversation is one-on-one or in a group, these conversations are vital to the well-being of our organizations, institutions, and communities, and persons of color living with health conditions.

For conversations on race to turn the tide of health in the African-American community, and to change and even save lives, they need to be handled with sensitivity. An awareness of the topic through race literacy is vital to the conversation, as is information about the continual stressors of racism in communities of color. It is important to allow the experiences garnered through the dialog to touch the heart of the providers. Information that touches the heart is vital to a race conversation. Acknowledging feelings are essential, along with the research and medical information. Race is emotional, personal, and institutional, and the daily impact of race on people of color takes its toll over a lifetime. Compassion and understanding are important when embarking on a conversation on race. The African-American community has a four-hundred-year history with intergenerational and historical trauma.

CHAPTER 3

INTERGENERATIONAL AND HISTORICAL TRAUMA

We do people a disservice when we separate emotions, mind, and spirit from the human body. America's history of race and racism, the traumatic events and experiences of African-Americans, and the intergenerational effects of these experiences should not be underestimated or ignored when dealing with the healthcare of these patients/clients. The history of African-Americans has been and continues to be brutal. From economy to psychology, from environmental racism to redlining, the continued violence perpetrated upon people of color takes its toll on their health and well-being. Moreover, the trauma of their violent history has been passed on from generation to generation without the benefit of healing, while mental health is mostly stigmatized in these communities. Add to that the micro-aggressions of everyday life and the extra stress becomes monumental.

In May 2016, *Teen Vogue* published an article on intergenerational trauma after many African-Americans commented that they would not watch the TV show *Roots* because they found it disturbing. There is a reason that African-Americans, who are descendants of enslaved persons might find the TV show Roots disturbing, and it's more than just the violent scenes.

Dr. Rachel Yehuda, professor of psychiatry at Icahn School of Medicine at Mount Sinai, has done extensive research on **epigenetics** and how trauma is passed on from one generation to another. She found that *"Serious incidents such as the Holocaust, slavery, create traumas that are passed on through shared family* *genes, through the generations."* In other words, our children inherit the genes affected by our trauma. In her work, Dr. Yehuda found that Holocaust survivors and Veterans of the Vietnam war who were suffering from PTSD had similar hormonal profiles. Africans and their descendants in the Americas and the Caribbean endured the trials of their enslavement for hundreds of years. Despite the trauma and continued injury, their resilience is nothing short of amazing. However, one can not ignore the possibility that these injuries, and the trauma passed down through the generations, may be affecting their health in ways that have yet to be explored.

In *Post Traumatic Slave Syndrome: America's Legacy of Enduring Injury and Healing,* Joy DeGruy writes about the effect of slavery on the African-American community:

"Parents feeling the need to protect their children from the police. Issues of skin color and hair texture continuing to dominate discussions regarding beauty and physical preference. The excessive focus on material

accumulation. People needing, wanting and dreaming, yet fearing they will not succeed. Most of all frustration. Frustration and anger, at times even rage, feelings that seem to dominate many of our lives. If you're black and living in America, none of this may be news to you."

While these behaviors were adapted in order to survive, continuing the behavior can be detrimental to a person's health, causing a consistent background layer of stress that underlies every day of a patient's/client's life, weakening their immune system.

Some patients/clients also suffer from secondary trauma caused by watching police beating and shooting African-Americans on TV or the web, watching the KKK marching on the streets, or even seeing the police stop a car as they drove past. What is normal to one person may be traumatic to others, causing them extra stress, which ultimately affects their health. Some people may be more vulnerable than others, depending on the amount of trauma they may have experienced in the past.

The racial disparities faced by people of color concerning the convenience (or inconvenience) of buying healthy food, access to green spaces, housing affordability and access, and wages (even for equal work) are part of the healthcare landscape. The microaggressions caused by implicit and explicit bias are also the cause of stress when dealing with store clerks and store security. Dealing with the police, dealing with difficult school systems (as children and then again as parents), and surviving family and community violence and a host of other situations that are beyond their control create daily stress that affects their health.

DISTRUST OF THE MEDICAL SYSTEM

Unethical medical practices have created distrust of the medical system. People of color fear that they will be experimented on or given experimental drugs without their consent. From the time of enslavement, African-Americans have been used as subjects for medical training. The Tuskegee experiment, sterilization to control populations, and the taking of HeLa cells for experiments, are a few of the best-known cases. But there are many cases which the reader can learn about by reading books such as *Medical Apartheid: The Dark History of Medical Experimentation on Black Americans from Colonial Times to the Present* by Harriet Washington.

CHAPTER 4
SELF-PREPARATION

Those speaking race in healthcare, need to know where they stand on the issue of race before entering the conversation. These questions might be helpful in becoming self-aware in preparation for the conversation:

- Is race something that affects individuals in the organization?
- Do you, as the one speaking, see race as someone else's problem?

- Does race affect you personally? If so, in what ways?
- Beyond the civil rights movement, how much do you know about race in America?

There are a lot of ways to prepare for a conversation on race. One can engage in race-related research about the past or the current state of the country. Information in journals and from reputable institutions, such as universities and think tanks, can prove very useful. Learning about American and particularly African-American history, beyond what was taught in the schools, is imperative. Assessing personal levels of comfort and discomfort with the topic of race can help see themselves see themselves as part of the conversation.

Personal experience with race as it relates to a particular work specialty is an added plus. Facts about how specific illnesses impact communities of color and the importance of retaining patients/clients in care is essential to the conversation. Bring an understanding of how stigma affects care to the conversation and a commitment to lifelong learning, humility, and curiosity. As a facilitator, be open to learning. The more conversations on race we engage in, the more we learn, the more comfortable we become with the topic, and the more creative ideas will be available.

The Journal of the National Medical Association states that "Clinicians providing care for African-Americans must bridge the racial divide and incorporate culturally relevant content in the health history. As an integral aspect of their professional growth, culturally competent healthcare providers must incorporate the idea of race consciousness in their work."

African-Americans, Native Americans, and people with language barriers have faced a long history of medical discrimination and experimentation. Again, the Journal of the National Medical Association states: "The atmosphere created by racial inferiority theories and stereotypes, 246 years of chattel slavery, along with biased educational processes, often led to medical and scientific abuse, unethical experimentation, and overutilization of African-Americans as subjects for teaching and training purposes."

In leading a conversation on race with a group of healthcare providers, the facilitator should take a few moments to breathe deeply with the participants. Conversations on race can be stressful, and two or three deep breaths can help participants relax. According to Harvard Health Publications, "One of the easiest ways to reduce stress is to simply focus your attention on your breath. You'll notice an immediate sense of relaxation that could help you relieve stress over time."

The breath unites us in ways that are immeasurable. Allow a sense of calm to be present. Experience the peace in the breath, and gently break the silence to start introductions. Allow all participants in the conversation the opportunity to say their names and to share whatever is in their hearts, as it relates to race and health equity. Remember that race in the healthcare conversation can save lives. The conversation is worth having.

CLARITY IS KEY

Clarity is gained through an honest appraisal of how the organization works with issues of race. An honest appraisal can help set an intention for the conversation. Is the conversation to look at race and its impact on organizational policy and how those policies may be affecting patients/clients? Is it to learn more about the patient/client? Is it to look at ways that historical trauma may be affecting patients/clients? Is it to address a specific issue in the community that is directly related to race and health? Is it a follow-up to a racial incident? Whatever the intention, the reason for coming together has been primarily to speak about race, so be clear about that from the start.

CONFRONTATION

Determine to maintain a nonconfrontational approach to the conversation. People often come to conversations on race with the warrior archetype active, locked and loaded. Confrontation is one of the ways that people use to resist the conversation. Facilitators of race conversations are expected to maintain their composure, while some participants may be looking to deny or deflect. As the lead in the conversation, participants will be looking to the facilitator to maintain an air of safety. Unless you feel confident in the conversation, it is best to bring in a skilled and experienced facilitator, especially if the organization is new at having conversations on race. The goal is to give healthcare providers information that enhances their awareness of the impact of race and racism on their patient's healthcare.

ALLOW THE PROCESS

Be prepared for the healing crisis, resistance, and hijackers. The best way to work with resistance is to acknowledge that it is difficult and even frightening to speak about race and that resistance is normal. Hijackers, on the other hand, are often acting out of a need for control, which comes from the anxiety caused by the conversation. This is why starting with deep breaths is important. Patience and deep breathing help to relieve stress and anxiety.

Even when people come to the conversation willingly, they are still carrying their unconscious biases about race. Especially when misunderstood because of the bias a listener may bring to the discussion, something that someone shares can become a trigger. A trigger is something that when heard, or experienced can throw the person emotionally off-kilter and can set off the fight, flight, or paralysis response. Maintain composure. People get triggered because they are carrying unprocessed internal pain, which manifests as ammunition that can explode when touched. Remain internally quiet and compassionately understanding, even when individuals in the group express pain and anger. Remember that authentic, kind, and caring responses can be disarming.

MAKE ROOM FOR THE UNEXPECTED

As the conversation on race begins, facilitators are encouraged to create a space of peace within themselves and make room for the unexpected. These conversations, while challenging, can be transformative, both individually and collectively. When we work on ourselves first, we learn our biases, gifts, and limitations. We learn to clear our inner pain and fill our hearts with peace and compassion. We begin to see our ignorance, denial, and anger, and we begin to heal. That healing allows us to become the light that lets all other lights shine. By sharing our story, we permit the other members of the group to tell their stories, creating a bond of safety that nurtures all those who are involved in the conversation. Having an experience of safety is very important to the conversation on race and health equity.

PREPARE FOR CRITICISM

While most of us don't want the responsibility of leading a conversation on race, we often have very particular ideas of what the conversation should be like and how it should be led. Don't let negativity be the light that guides.

We can prepare to be effective conveners of conversations on race and health equity by:
- Doing research and gathering facts, such as:
  - Historical facts
  - Information about the effects of race on the health of communities of color
  - How race affects the way organizations serve people of color
- Honoring and allowing emotions
- Being honest about how the organization works with issues of race
- Becoming less judgmental
- Allowing time for processing new information

Build processing time into the conversation. "Processing" is more than just trying to make sense of information. It means taking in information and allowing it to move through the mind, body, spirit, and emotions. Processing allows for the catharsis that can come from a new realization and leads to new ways of being.

CHAPTER 5
THE SETUP

Before beginning a conversation on race, it is imperative to realize that the daily realities of people of color and whites are very different in our nation. Participants in these conversations are apt to differ in their views, opinions, and beliefs about the American experience. It is, therefore, vital for you as the facilitator to listen and share from your personal experience and that of your patients/clients.

A Manual for a New Dialogue

WHERE IS THE CONVERSATION TAKING PLACE?

Is it in an organization or an institution? Is it in a community setting or a town hall meeting? Is the conversation a one on one, with another healthcare provider or a patient? Where the conversation takes place, and the number of people attending will determine the structure of that conversation. Keep in mind that smaller groups (six to twelve participants) are more manageable than larger groups. When working with a town hall type of gathering, it's best to have approximately one facilitator for every ten participants.

THE PURPOSE

A successful race conversation offers facts for the head and experiences for the heart. Without the experiential work that touches the heart, a conversation on race becomes another academic exercise — a lot of great information but none of the experiences that lead to transformation. Prepare to show part of a documentary or to engage the group in a meaningful experience. The race-history exercise in this manual has proved to be meaningful for over a decade.

To have a successful conversation on race, all parties should come to the table with some sense of their biases and prejudices and should be open to uncovering new ones. This does not only apply to whites. People of color were also raised with the same prejudices as whites and need to garda gains their own internalized racial conditioning. Conscious awareness of our personal history with race and our personal triggers can set the foundation for growth and understanding. It helps us decipher feelings and emotions, and it uncovers reasons that we react the way we do around the subject of race.

Knowing our background and history, including family history with the topic, can go a long way in helping us stay present with what is happening in the conversation at any given point. We need our history for healing and transformation.

BE CLEAR ABOUT THE PURPOSE OF THE CONVERSATION

What is the purpose of the conversation? Is it to teach, to learn, to persuade or to negotiate? Is it to share, to understand, or to process emotions after a traumatic event? Is the purpose of the conversation to grieve a loss, to create an action plan? Is it for fact-finding or informing? Is it to find out about a patient's racial backgrounds or stressors? We need to get clear about the purpose because the purpose will drive the direction of the conversation.

FOLLOW-UP

Follow-up is very important. Conversations on race create new questions about ourselves, our work, and our lives. They awaken memories and experiences long forgotten; this is where follow-up can be helpful, especially if the original group remains intact after the original conversation. Having people with whom we have had a shared experience gives us the opportunity to express without feeling judged and opens the door to exponential growth and learning. Planning for three or more conversations lets the participants know that they will not be left alone with whatever the experience awakens in them.

A Manual for a New Dialogue

CHAPTER 6
RULES OF ENGAGEMENT

The rules of engagement are the ground rules that help us create a safe space for participants to share their experiences. They are the cornerstone of the conversation and give us a place to return to should we get lost in the process. These ground rules include rules for speaking and for listening. They are about respecting the experiences of all participants and about allowing the expression of all feelings and emotions. They also are about reminding participants that everyone is responsible for his or her feelings and emotions. This means that if what we hear in the conversation is awakening feelings in us, we cannot blame others for those feelings with statements such as "You make me angry." A more accurate statement would be "What I heard makes me feel angry." The difference between these two statements is that the previous gives away our power by allowing others to "make us" angry. The latter is nonaccusatory and keeps the responsibility, and therefore the power, with the individual. And the rules are about guaranteeing the anonymity of any participant who wants it.

These conversations are not set up to blame, point a finger, or accuse anyone of wrongdoing. Rather they are for informing, sharing, and expressing thoughts and feelings in an environment of compassion and care, and offering new and creative ideas. Setting ground rules for sharing and listening can go a long way towards making speakers feel heard and towards giving space for the listeners to process what they are hearing. Keep in mind that even with the ground rules, emotions may escalate as people express long-held views and forgotten experiences. While feelings of anger, resentment, and frustration will arise, it is important that these feelings not be taken out on our colleagues; race has enough pain and trauma attached to it. Determine to be a non-violent expression of healing by choosing compassion instead of judgment. Listen, hear, feel. The truth about race is painful, no matter which way we turn it. Using words that express feelings helps to put things in perspective. The section on emotions includes the Center for Nonviolent Communication Feelings Inventory to help us get clear about how we feel.

Here are twenty rules for sharing that you may find helpful. It is suggested that a copy of the rules you select and the feelings inventory be given to each participant.

THE RULES FOR SHARING

1. Make room for silence, even when it is uncomfortable.
2. Sharing is voluntary.
3. Everything shared here remains here.
4. Everyone gets an opportunity to express his or her views.

A Manual for a New Dialogue

5. Respect the experience and knowledge of all participants.
6. Listen with an open heart and an open mind.
7. Do not roll your eyes to signal feelings and opinions to other participants.
8. Be aware of resistance from self and others.
9. No hijacking the conversation.
10. Make "I" statements: "I think," "I feel."
11. No talking while others are sharing.
12. No sidebar conversations.
    13. Allow participants to emote.
    14. Allow personal feelings.
    15. Allow for the feelings of others.
    16. Stay open to the experience.
    17. Allow for change and transformation.
    18. Quiet the inner voices.
    19. Avoid finger-pointing.
    20. Make eye contact.

It is not necessary to use all of the above statements. Feel free to pick some and add additional ones that are appropriate to the group being led. Always remember that racism is an inherited dysfunction and people don't know what they don't know. Compassion is needed for all involved.

QUESTIONS TO CONSIDER

When having an important conversation, what rules of engagement are most important?

What makes participants feel unsafe in a conversation on race?

What makes participants feel safe in a conversation on race?

CREATING A SAFE SPACE

Conversations about race are sensitive. They are important and can be precursors to change. How we set up the conversation and how we conduct ourselves makes a vast difference in our ability to effect change. It is also important to understand the intention behind our words. When a conversation necessarily elicits painful memories and painful experiences, how we broach that conversation determines how successful it will be. Race can be a "toxic" topic, as it is harsh, and can be, in many ways, a life changer. It can also be emotional as mentioned earlier. For a race conversation to be successful, those engaged it must create a safe space for all the participants. The above rules can be helpful in creating that space of safety. Remember that even with our best intentions and planning, there may still be those who feel threatened and unsafe during the experience.

PERSONAL HISTORY WITH RACE

Everyone has a race history — even the person who says, "My first experience with someone of a different race was when I went to college." That's that person's history and experience! It's not good or bad, right or wrong. It just is. Each person's history is important, and coming to the conversation with an awareness of one's personal history with race can go a long way in understanding whatever reactions and feelings arise during the conversation. It can also help us keep track of our triggers, and it can help us get a sense of where we are stuck and why, as well as feel where the emotions are lodged in our bodies. To understand where the emotions are in your body, notice if there is tightness or discomfort in your body when speaking about race. Try to pinpoint where the discomfort is. Are your fists tight? Is there a knot in your stomach? Are your jaws tight? Is your mouth dry? Notice any bodily sensations; the information the body gives is very telling.

ENCOUNTERING DIFFERENCES

A study done by the Pew Research Center in 2016 shows a significant difference in perceptions of racial fairness. African-American and white participants were asked how blacks were treated relative to whites by the police, the court system, in stores and restaurants, in the workplace, in public schools, when applying for a mortgage, and dealing with the healthcare system.

According to the study, the percentage saying that blacks are treated less fairly varies widely. These numbers come directly from the Pew Research Center.

Percent of each group saying blacks are treated worse than whites in each context

CONTEXT	WHITES	BLACKS
Police encounters	50%	84%
Courts	43%	75%
Loan applications	25%	66%
Public education	15%	51%
Workplaces	22%	64%
Stores and restaurants	21%	49%
Voting	20%	43%

This list is just the tip of the iceberg. Be prepared to encounter all sorts of differences and to learn how even your closest friends have been affected by this thing we call race.

PREPARE FOR OVERTIME

While race is not one of those conversations, people typically jump to attend, when they start talking about race they find that they have a great deal to say. For some, their years of silence create a need to speak at length when they find an audience willing to listen to them, so the conversation can easily run beyond the time allotted; nevertheless, watch the time. Give everyone an opportunity to speak, and, if someone wants to continue the conversation beyond the time allocated, do what you can to honor this need by offering to stay a few additional minutes, if y can. Close the conversation by letting others know that the time for this conversation is now over, and those who choose to stay may do so. Offer to email the time and date for the follow-up conversation.

A Manual for a New Dialogue

CHAPTER 7

HISTORY

Everyone and everything has a history. As each moment passes into the next, that which is, becomes what was. Regardless of how we amass that history, it is personal, and it becomes part of what we carry into our conversations.

None of us was born with the awareness of race as a separating factor between humans. It was something we learned from our environment and from our circle of influence, which is made up of the family, community, corporate and private systems, politics, media, peers, and the placement of what we call home, be it urban, suburban, or rural. Our circle of influence helps to form our worldview. And our worldview forms the filters through which we experience life.

Our history is an array of experiences colored by our emotions, whether they are positive or negative, intense or less so. Our history forms our character and determines how we will act in a given moment or a particular situation. Our history becomes a protective shield that we hide behind. And, unless we have conscious awareness of that history, it can run our lives. When it comes to race, everyone has a history. Whether that history is that we were raised in a homogeneous community or we were raised by liberal parents who believed that racism was wrong, we nevertheless have some connection to race in America. And this is where our conversation begins because racism is personal as much as it is collective, historical, and institutional. Our history is an important part of what we bring to the conversation.

So, what did we learn about race? What did we learn from our parents, other adults, the media, our school, and our peers? Was race included in or omitted from the conversation at home and at school? Did we receive positive or negative information about race relations? What was the racial makeup of the people in our town, our school, and our family? Who were our heroes growing up? Were there any heroes in our lives who did not look like us? Who were the people featured in paintings at our museums? Did they look like us? Who were the stars in our movies? Did they look like us? Did both our parents go to college? Did they own their home? Did we go on summer vacations, to summer camp, or music school? Did our school get brand new books every year? Did our school have computers, a swimming pool, a ski club, and international travel? Did we have access to green spaces when we were a child? Do we remember our first experience with race? I purposely did not want to give these questions categories; rather, I want them to represent the rambling of the mind as we begin to uncover the layers of our racial conditioning.

Answering all of these questions is important because we bring ourselves to any conversation on race, and it's essential for us to know ourselves within the context of race. What bothers us and even frightens us about a conversation on race? Do we feel we might be called out, called a name, be accused of something? Does the conversation bring up feelings of anger, shame, guilt, mistrust, culpability or disconnection? Examine those feelings and be aware what feelings you bring into the conversation as part of your background.

Just as human beings have a history, so do events. For instance, did the organization attempt to have conversations on race before? How did those conversations go? That information can be critical in addressing why participants may not want to participate in the new attempt. It is helpful to understand that history to come to the conversation prepared to have a successful exchange. Those who come to the conversation may have personal experience with the event in question, and their reactions will be based on that. As facilitators, we do not know the breadth of experiences our participants bring. When it comes to race, people are at various levels of awareness and experience. Situations in which people are grieving the loss of a loved one due to some racial incident, need to be navigated with compassion and care.

A Manual for a New Dialogue

CHAPTER 8

EXPERIENCE
Something That Touches the Heart

I have heard it said that the heart measures time by experiences. If this is so, some of us are older than our years. In my seminars, I use film to create experiences that touch the hearts of the participants. Film offers visual content that stimulates the imagination and helps illustrate another's life experience. Film can illustrate what it's like to have been enslaved on a plantation, bringing forth feelings of restriction, oppression, and loss of freedom. Unless we are a person of color, we are not going to know what racial oppression feels like, but we may have an awareness of what bullying feels like, what loss and grief feel like, and what not fitting in feels like. We may also know what it feels like to not be safe, not be welcomed, or not belong. Now imagine these experiences becoming a lifestyle, where everything in life is colored by those painful experiences, and as if that were not enough, the country has institutionalized our pain.

There are countless daily slights that accrue over time. When we are passed over for promotion time and time again; when a store clerk asks everyone else in the store if they need help, but doesn't ask us; when a valet acts as if we are invisible and assists a customer who arrived after us. These slights are stressful and take a mental and physical toll on people of color. Accrued over a lifetime, these stresses affect the physical body. Moreover, many people of color have a subtle sense of never feeling safe that also adds to the constant state of stress.

We all know that living in today's world can be stressful. But when we add to that the daily pressure of being a person of color, particularly if we have a significant amount of melanin in our skin, we create a situation that can go as far as affecting our health. Race affects people of color from birth to death, and in some cases, being black can begin to affect us even before birth. Take, for instance, what the Centers for Disease Control and Prevention has to say about pregnancy, childbirth, and infant mortality rates: "Infants of non-Hispanic black women had the highest mortality rates from low birth weight. The rate for non-Hispanic black women was 2.5 times that of non-Hispanic white women."

The CDC also says that "pregnancy-related health outcomes are influenced by factors such as race, ethnicity, age, and income, but most importantly — a woman's health."

Interestingly enough, next to the CDC article is an advertisement that reads, "Get healthy before you get pregnant." While it's not impossible, it's hard to be healthy in an environment of racial discrimination and racial bias. If we are to have a healthy society, we need to think of health as related to the whole being; we have to consider daily stressors, physical environment, historical and intergenerational trauma, economic positioning, and countless other nuances that make up the experiences of an individual.

According to *Unnatural Causes: Is Inequality Making Us Sick*, a documentary produced by California News Reel, "It turns out there's much more to our health than bad habits, healthcare, or unlucky genes. The social conditions in which we are born, live, and work profoundly affect our well-being and longevity."

"When the Bough Breaks," a 28-minute segment, is part of the four-hour documentary. It focuses on infant mortality rates as well as on preterm (under 37 weeks) and low birth-weight babies. In it, we learn that "researchers are circling in on the added burden of racism through the life-course as a long-term risk factor."

The episode notes that "African-American women with graduate degrees still face a greater risk of delivering pre-term, low birth-weight babies than white women who didn't finish high school."

The CDC notes that the infant-mortality "rate is often used as an indicator to measure the health and well-being of a nation because factors affecting the health of entire populations can also impact the mortality rate of infants."

Beyond diet and exercise, life-course stress has been found to be a significant factor affecting heart disease, diabetes, obesity, and ultimately longevity. Patients/clients with diagnoses of HIV and AIDS also face the stigma of their disease, sexual stigma and in many cases, sexual-orientation stigma. LGBTQ patients/clients are often discriminated against and bullied by our society, their own family members, and at times even their healthcare providers. A survey covered in *LGBTQ Nation* showed that 29 percent of gay or bisexual African-American men had encountered stigma in healthcare, and 48 percent mistrusted medical institutions.

The reasons were previously mentioned in this manual. The life-course stress faced by people of color is enough to cause healthcare concerns. Consider this, when treating African-Americans you are not just treating their present health concern, you are also treating life-course stress, intergenerational and historical trauma, and the underlying internal and subconscious stress that comes with that.

The phrase "post-traumatic stress disorder" implies that the stress is in the past. African-Americans in the US suffer from what could be called "constant-traumatic stress disorder," and it affects their health and well-being. However, external forces, which are constantly at play in their lives, such as being stopped, in some cases harassed and even killed by the police while driving. Being followed in the stores, being ignored in the boardroom, getting lower pay for the same work, being passed over for promotion, being profiled while walking down a street, and other forms of disrespect, take their toll over a lifetime. Healthcare workers assisting African-American patients/clients could benefit those they serve by providing trauma-informed care.

Speaking race to have healthier communities of color means bringing awareness of life-course stress and its impact on the health of patients/clients. When we come together to speak about our experiences with race, we need to remember that while we live in a country of "equality," our experiences are far from equal. The life-course stress carried by people of color is an added stress their white counterparts are spared. At the same time, it takes great courage and strength to live and thrive under systems of oppression, where institutional racism and personal racial bias are the norm.

The toll that racism takes on people of color has a widespread impact on the health of the community. We see it in higher incidences of high blood pressure, diabetes, and countless other illnesses. From birth to death, people of color face odds and stressors that their white counterparts do not.

Daniel J. DeMoon, a writer with WebMD, writes that *"Several deadly diseases strike black Americans harder and more often than they do white Americans."* We've all seen the statistics for African-Americans, who suffer higher incidents of lung scarring, diabetes, limb amputation, kidney disease, asthma. While Black men have lower exposure to tobacco, they are 50% more likely to die of lung cancer. The Black community has younger men and women with high blood pressure than their white counterparts, and they have higher cancer deaths.

For some whites, the awareness of having the odds fixed in their favor, without their consent or request, brings up feelings of culpability, shame, and fear. Their fragility around the topic of race and their power to create laws and change the lives of people of color make them dangerous in the eyes of many. Whites carry an internalized fear of revolt that is rarely if ever discussed. This unconscious and mostly unmentioned fear has led to over-policing and over-incarceration of nonwhite populations and, in particular, African-Americans and Latinos.

Coming to a conversation about a topic that brings up these feelings isn't easy. Finding out that things are not as equal as one might have thought is jarring to the belief system and can throw one into cognitive dissonance. That's not comfortable! However, hiding from the truth of how our collective history still affects us doesn't heal us. To the contrary, it keeps us trapped in cycles of repetition. We all need to join the conversation to find out what we don't know and to work together to transform our collective situation. Lives are at stake.

As we encounter difficult moments in facilitating the conversation, remember to *breathe*. Breath is flowing life, and when we breathe, we bring the flow of life into those places within us that were lifeless or stuck. Breathe slowly and deliberately. Breathe into the parts of the body that have the discomfort.

More often than not, it's not the conversation that makes us feel uncomfortable. If we are experiencing discomfort, the discomfort was already there. All the conversation did was bring it to the surface. The good news is that we now have a new awareness and that awareness gives us choice. We can choose to accept what we learned about ourselves; we can choose to remain unchanged by the awareness, or we can choose to change it. Choice is power. It takes a lot of energy to hold the discomfort of internalized pain in place, especially if it was so deep inside of us that we didn't realize it was there. Denial does not heal. But awareness can, because of the power of choice.

As facilitators of conversations on race, we will need to give our participants experiences that bring awareness of their history with race, as well as some awareness of the racial biases they carry. Use research, film, and other media to bring home the point. Be patient and be compassionate. Remember that people don't know what they don't know and that they are often not aware of their biases.

BIAS IN THE CONVERSATION

In "Implicit Bias and the American Juror," Jennifer K. Elek and Paula Hannaford-Agor refer to both explicit and implicit bias. "Explicit bias," they explain, is "the form of bias that a person intentionally endorses (and the traditional definition of racial prejudice that most people recognize)." Implicit bias, by contrast, operates without self-awareness and affects our understanding, leads to judgments and influences our perception and behavior toward others."

Racial bias can be exhibited in organizations in the form of microaggressions, such as leaving certain members of the organization out of a meeting or a conversation; judging people's intelligence by the color of their skin, the sound of their voice, and even their accent. Deciding not to share information with someone in the organization or a patient/client because of the belief that that person will not understand or will misuse the information. Not seeking input from certain members of the organization because they are perceived as aggressive, flippant, or uppity; or taking a "we don't need input from the help" attitude and not consulting the employees who are interacting with the people that are being served.

We all have biases. They are part of the human condition. Our biases are meant to keep us safe. However, not all biases are racial, institutionalized, and supported through a lifetime of social propaganda. Being self-reflective and examining one's personal biases is important to bringing clarity to the conversation on race. Awareness of one's biases is essential to understanding how and why one gets triggered. On the next page, you will find a quick bias test that facilitators can use to help themselves, and their participants become aware of their internalized conditioning.

A QUICK BIAS TEST

Try this quick bias test with your participants.

Time: 20 Minutes

Supplies: Pen and Paper

The purpose of the test is to bring awareness of our unquestioned, biased, assumptions in everyday life.

Instructions

Ask participants write down the first thing that comes to mind. Don't think about the answer, get a quick visual and write the description of who you see in your mind's eye on the piece of paper.

What is the first picture that pops into your head, when you hear the following?

1. a scientist
2. an agricultural worker
3. a mom with four children
4. a homeless person
5. a CEO
6. the Board Chair

7. a social worker
8. a kindergarten teacher
9. an astronaut
10. a garbage collector
11. an art collector

Once participants are finished writing their descriptions, go through each of the descriptions, and ask the participants to share their answers. Encourage participants to speak about the race of the person they imagined. There are no wrong answers with this test. Then ask participants if they have ever questioned these assumptions.

Next, ask participants if they ever find themselves being racially biased. As the facilitator, you can start the conversation by giving an example out of your own experience.

CHAPTER 9

RACE IN THE HEALTHCARE ORGANIZATION

Race affects everything in the organization, from who serves on the board of directors to who receives services and the even the quality of those services. How does race show up in your healthcare organization? Look around the organization and ask these questions.

1. Is the organization serving people of color?

2. Are there people of color represented in decision-making?
3. Who is included in or left out of important conversations?
4. Who speaks up about race in the organization?
5. Are people who speak about race supported by management or their peers?
6. Is the board comfortable with the race conversation?
7. Are there people of color who are department heads in the organization?
8. Are there members of the board who are people of color?
9. Does the organization develop programs without input from the community?
10. Does the organization ask the community what it needs?
11. How does the organization get the word to the community about its services?
12. Does the organization only measure resources in dollars and cents, or in human capital, such as talents, ability, and experiences?
13. Does the organization believe that LGBTQ people can't be racist?

14. Does the organization have a strong relationship with the community? If not, what steps can be taken to strengthen relationships with the community?
15. Are all of the patients/clients given information about what services are available to them?
16. Does the organization tell all patients/clients what medications and procedures are available to them?
17. Does the organization let the color of patients'/clients' skin or their accent determine what information it will share and what to make available to them?
18. Is the organization communicating across disciplines and departments?
19. Do the members of the organization consult only with pockets of inner circles?
20. Is the organization communicating in a way that is socio-economically, educationally, and racially inclusive?

This last question is about addressing the barriers that separate coworkers at different levels within the organization and keep communication from flowing smoothly. If any of these questions highlights a problem at an organization, then that organization could benefit from having conversations on race facilitated by a professional. As the facilitator, keep these questions in mind going into the conversation.

WHAT IS AFFECTED IN THE ORGANIZATION?

Race affects all levels of service in an organization. It affects:

- recruitment
- hiring
- salary
- promotions
- mentoring
- trust
- field-based outreach
- counseling and peer counseling
- treatment and care
- case management
- support groups
- communication
- partnering with organizations

- resources
- referral and support services
- access to organizational information
- policies and procedures
- ... and so much more.

Ultimately the persons who are hurt the most by this are the very people the organization was created to serve, the patients/clients.

Having an awareness of the role that race plays in a healthcare organization and how it affects members of the organization across the board is vital to the conversation. Being able to speak about race in our organizations with an understanding of how race affects all departments and areas is very important. If the intention is to be an agent of change in the community, then the organizations may need to model that change for the community by creating an equitable workplace that speaks openly about race. Getting comfortable with the uncomfortable conversation and its effect on the entire organization can be a lifesaver.

Speaking Race in Healthcare

CHAPTER 10

COMPONENTS OF THE CONVERSATION

TELLING

Our stories are important parts of us. They capture the essence of our experiences. Sometimes, though, they get muddled with our emotions, and it becomes hard to distinguish between fact and fiction. Our stories become a mixture of what happened, how we felt at the moment, and what meaning we attached to events that happened. For instance, imagine being a small child in school. The teacher asks a question, but you do not know the answer. Here is one way that the experience may be processed:

1) <u>Fact</u>: The teacher asked a question, and you did not have the answer.

2) <u>Feeling</u>: You felt uncomfortable and inadequate at that moment.

3) <u>Meaning attached to the experience</u>: You may think of yourself as not being as smart as the other children in the class. You may think that the teacher believes you not to be as intelligent as the other children in the class. You may believe that you will never be a successful student.

The feelings that arise while these thoughts swirl around are feelings of inadequacy, discomfort, isolation, disconnection, shame, tension, and anxiety, to name a few. These negative emotions surrounding our memory of the event can act as the dragon guarding the actual memory of the original event. When we are unwilling to face the dragon of our emotions, we stay stuck in a cycle of repetition. While we can see the possibility of a new future, we are unable to move toward it.

By unpacking our stories, separating facts from emotions and the meanings we have given our experiences, we become clear and can speak from the heart. Being able to state what happened without embellishments keeps things clear, without ignoring the feelings that our experiences or those of others evoke in us. On the contrary, stating how an experience makes us feel is very important and keeps us from blaming others for our personal feelings. Telling our stories makes us vulnerable, and for people who are already wounded, or fragile, that can be difficult. However, telling our stories in a safe and supportive environment can be liberating. When we share our stories, the burden lightens.

More often than not, there are two parts to a story: the facts of what happened and the story we build around those facts. The story we build acts like a wall that keeps us safe, but at the same time, it keeps us separate, it's important to be conscious of that. We spend a great deal of time defending our stories, and we use them to justify behaviors that do not serve us.

QUESTIONS TO CONSIDER

What story do we tell about race in America?

Do we ever speak about our personal race history?

How do we tell our story of race? Is it through

- facts
- feelings and emotions
- meaning attached
- all of the above

QUESTIONS TO CONSIDER

Does our organization tell its story of race?

Does our story of race play out in our interactions with coworkers and patients/clients?

What do we tell our family and friends about race in the organization?

To dismantle racism in your organization, we first have to get comfortable speaking about race.

CHAPTER 11

LISTENING AND HEARING

Listening is an art. Like any art worth mastering, it takes practice.

Listening is something we do all the time. Listening is an action. It's giving one's attention to a sound. We do it so much that sometimes we listen without hearing, as when someone is speaking to us and what they are saying is not registering with us. Hearing is perceiving sound or auditory perceptions. There are also times when we hear or perceive sound without actively trying to listen. An example is when we happen upon an existing conversation and hear something not intended for us, such as a racial joke we were not supposed to hear. However, when listening and hearing are combined with an open heart and an open mind, the experience can be transformative.

Facing the speaker, making eye contact, and having a posture of attention creates a momentary bond between speaker and listener. If this bond is nurtured, it can lead to even deeper sharing. To listen and hear with an open mind and an open heart is to create a supportive space for sharing our stories.

In my "Race Demystified" seminars, I ask participants how they feel after engaging in a listening exercise. More often than not they say, "I felt heard." Feeling heard keeps us from needing to repeat ourselves. Feeling heard makes us feel cared for and nurtured, and it makes us feel that we are important and that we count.

Listening is paying attention. Listening works best when we can quiet our inner voices and can allow the voice of the other to penetrate our being and open us up. But most often, what we hear is filtered through our own life experiences and memories — what we know and believe about a topic, and what we have heard or have seen as it relates to the matter. We even bring our lack of information to our experience of listening. And when it comes to the topic of race, we have many gaps in our knowledge and a great deal of misinformation.

Listening and hearing are choices we make. And how we hear determines how we process the information we receive. We can listen through our anger and pain. We can listen through our connection or our compassion. We can listen through the voices of the past or the stillness of the present, but, regardless of how we listen, what we hear will determine how we react.

Deep listening requires that we suspend ourselves, our personalities, and what we believe for a moment by stopping the mind from wandering to places like what to cook for dinner, or what to get from the grocery store. It requires that we stop analyzing the speaker or falling into judgment. Deep listening is about creating a quiet space within us that allows the other person's words to echo back to them. In that echo, they hear their own stories and feel their pain. Deep listening lets us "feel" peoples' body language as they express in silence something for which they have no words. In short, deep listening is a practice that can help us to see ourselves in the mirror of the other and vice-versa. As a listener, we become a comforting agent and a healing balm.

QUESTIONS TO CONSIDER

When someone says racism, what do we hear?

What have we heard about race in our organization?

Do we feel ourselves shutting down the moment we hear the word race?

What do we hear when someone speaks of white privilege?

CHAPTER 12
QUESTIONING

Questions are important to conversations. Questions help with understanding and sometimes lead to more questions. However, questions can also be used to change the conversation. How we ask questions and what questions we choose to ask determine the direction a conversation about race will take. To keep the conversation moving in the direction of the goal, there are certain things facilitators need to keep in mind.

HIJACKING

Be aware of how participants hijack conversations by asking certain questions when they are uncomfortable. One way a participant may hijack the conversation is to ask inappropriate questions about someone's personal life, or questions that have nothing to do with the subject at hand.

RESISTANCE

Resistance to the conversation can show up in a variety of ways, such as checking out mentally or emotionally. Resistance can look like giving more attention to the voices in the head than to the voice of the person speaking, such as going into mental judgment of the speaker (i.e., Brenda is not very smart); not giving other participants the opportunity to speak; or interrupting.

In my seminars, I engage participants in a particular exercise of listening where they are not allowed to ask questions. While some listeners might find it uncomfortable, the speaker who gets to speak without interruption feels heard.

Still, questions are important for clarification. They can also act as an intervention and can be useful in the process of healing. The right question at the right time can make all the difference in our understanding of the topic at hand. Questions such as, "Can we be more specific and share more detail about this topic?" "How does that make us feel?" and "Did that remind us of a specific incident?" may prove valuable.

Before asking questions, take a moment to examine your motives. Ask questions that are open-ended, and that contain within them a desire to know more about the speaker or the subject. Be introspective and breathe for a minute with the questions before you ask them. Sometimes that kind of pause allows for a moment of clarity in which we see the answer to the question within the question itself. It also allows us to be in touch with our feelings.

Speaking Race in Healthcare

CHAPTER 13

EMOTIONS

Processing, in this case, is for healing and transformation.

Most of us are pretty "heady." We need facts and figures to determine whether something is worth our time or to discern whether what we are hearing is right or wrong. The problem is that, as mentioned earlier in this manual, race is emotional as much as it is personal and institutional. We can't solve the problems of the heart by simply using our heads. We need a combination of both head and heart to make the transformation needed in our racialized nation. We need it to see the intersections of race, health, and the higher incidents of disease in communities of color.

Emotions need to be processed. Processing can happen quickly, or it can take days, weeks, or even months as the information passes through the filters of our awareness. Processing emotions is not necessarily about thinking things through. It is more about allowing the information to filter through to the subconscious mind, where we might even receive a new awareness. We can take information and try to make sense of it, mull it around in our heads. But, if we truly want it to transform us, then it needs that ten-inch drop into the heart, where we carry our deepest feelings. There it can take its proper place. If need be, we might even allow ourselves to be vulnerable enough for the information to break our hearts so that the light of new awareness can get in and heal us from the inside out.

In some cultures, "never let them see you cry" is a motto for many people. We want to avoid painful emotions; we often hide from our feelings. But, when it comes to race, emotions spill over into our conversations and even onto our streets, as conversations about race become tense and peaceful protests turn into rioting. We feel anger, fear, disconnection, isolation, oppression, guilt, shame, and much more. E-motion is moving energy and is sometimes referred to as energy in motion. Emotions move us, especially if we are stuck, from where we were to where we could be.

We like things in nice, neat, predictable packages. But feelings and emotions are often unpredictable. Since race is a scary subject, to begin with, the thought of adding emotions makes the topic even more frightening. So, when it comes to race, we are very good at intellectualizing the subject, while living in denial of its damaging effects. We are experts at quoting numbers, percentages, and ratios. When it comes to race, we have more research than we can read in one lifetime. We have been studying race and researching people of color since the first Africans were brought to the New World as free laborers. But all of that science and research means little if we don't allow our humanity to be touched by the information, and transform us from the inside out. Feelings are important; they are attached to our needs.

The following is a list of feelings from Nonviolent Communications. This list is included to help us give words to our feelings. It is a useful list to share with participants, and as facilitators, we can use this list to clarify our feelings. The following is a list, copied with permission from the Nonviolent Communications website (NVC).

CHAPTER 14

FEELINGS INVENTORY

FEELINGS WHEN NEEDS ARE SATISFIED

Feelings Inventory copied with permission from the Website: **www.cnvc.org** Email: **cnvc@cnvc.org** Phone: (505) 244-4041. Copied with permission

AFFECTIONATE
compassionate
friendly
loving
open-hearted
sympathetic
tender
warm

ENGAGED
absorbed
alert
curious
engrossed
enchanted
entranced
fascinated
interested
intrigued
involved
spellbound
stimulated

HOPEFUL
expectant
encouraged
optimistic

CONFIDENT
empowered
open
proud
safe
secure

EXCITED
amazed
animated
ardent
aroused
astonished
dazzled
eager
energetic
enthusiastic
giddy
invigorated
lively
passionate
surprised
vibrant

GRATEFUL
appreciative
moved
thankful
touched

INSPIRED
amazed
awed
wonder

JOYFUL
amused
delighted
glad
happy
jubilant
pleased
tickled

REFRESHED
enlivened
rejuvenated
renewed
rested
restored
revived

PEACEFUL
calm
clear-headed
comfortable
centered
content
equanimous
fulfilled
mellow
quiet
relaxed
relieved
satisfied
serene
still
tranquil
trusting

EXHILARATED
blissful
ecstatic
elated
enthralled
exuberant
radiant
rapturous
thrilled

FEELINGS WHEN NEEDS ARE NOT SATISFIED

AFRAID
apprehensive
dread
foreboding
frightened
mistrustful
panicked
petrified
scared
suspicious
terrified
wary
worried

ANNOYED
aggravated
dismayed
disgruntled
displeased
exasperated
distracted
impatient
irritated
irked

ANGRY
enraged
furious
incensed
indignant
irate
livid
outraged
resentful

AVERSION
animosity
appalled
contempt
disgusted
dislike
hate
horrified
hostile
repulsed

VULNERABLE
fragile
guarded
insecure
sensitive
helpless

CONFUSED
ambivalent
baffled
bewildered
dazed
hesitant
lost
mystified
perplexed
puzzled
torn

DISCONNECTED
alienated
aloof
apathetic
bored
cold
detached
distant
indifferent
numb
removed
uninterested
withdrawn

DISQUIET
agitated
alarmed
discombobulated
disconcerted
disturbed
perturbed
rattled
restless
shocked
startled
surprised
troubled
turbulent
turmoil
uncomfortable
uneasy
unnerved
unsettled
upset

EMBARRASSED
ashamed
chagrined
flustered
guilty

FATIGUE
beat
burnt out
depleted
exhausted
lethargic
listless
sleepy
tired
weary
worn out

PAIN
agony
anguished
bereaved
devastated
grief
heartbroken
hurt
lonely
miserable
regretful
remorseful

SAD
depressed
dejected
despair
despondent
disappointed
discouraged
disheartened
forlorn
gloomy
heavy hearted
hopeless
melancholy
unhappy
wretched

TENSE
anxious
cranky
distressed
distraught
edgy
fidgety
frazzled
irritable
jittery

NOTES

While books can give us a great deal of information and can enhance our awareness by giving us some of the data we hadn't known, that data still needs to be processed through our emotions. We cannot solve with our heads an issue that's centered in our hearts. Make no mistake about it: race is emotional and personal. And when we bravely enter the heart to deal with it, it is there we encounter the healing crisis.

The crisis happens because where we are now is different from where we are headed. To get to this new place, we have to shed what we are holding in the present. In other words, we have to release what is familiar and live with uncertainty, at least for a while. As the French author, André Gide wisely wrote, "One does not discover new lands without consenting to lose sight of the shore for a very long time."

QUESTIONS TO CONSIDER

As you look at the CNVC Feelings Inventory what feelings best describe our relationship to race?

How comfortable are you with your feelings and emotions?

How comfortable are you with the feelings and emotions of others when it comes to race?

How emotional do you believe Americans are about race?

Speaking Race in Healthcare

CHAPTER 15

THE HEALING CRISIS

There is no greater chaos than that which happens when we choose to heal.

The road to healing and transformation is fraught with chaos and upheaval. Detoxing from our racialized ways can cause cognitive dissonance and throw us into crisis. Things often seem worst, because we see the toxicity everywhere. Sometimes feelings of hopelessness surface, we want to get back to not knowing, but we know that we can't. To get where we are headed (a place of greater wholeness), we need to leave the past behind, and for many, that is not easy. One dictionary defines a crisis as, "an emotionally significant event or radical change of status in a person's life; the turning point for better or worse in an acute disease; an unstable or crucial time or state of affairs in which a decisive change is impending."[i] Some may feel as if everything they learned about race was a lie or may have a hard time believing the experiences of others. For some, learning about race in America may cause inconsistencies with what they learned and believed.

The more we learn about race, the more difficult it becomes to have conversations with the people in our lives who have not been exposed to the same information. When we try to share what we have learned, we may find it difficult to explain our experience. Moreover, those who we try to share with may also have a hard time with the information and may do their best to avoid the conversation.

When it comes to race, many people feel as if they've heard it all before, till they engage in conversation and suddenly are faced with a country they didn't know existed and with people they believed were having an equal experience to their own. An example of this occurred in New Orleans with Hurricane Katrina:

"Hurricane Katrina exposed the shocking extent to which poverty and income disparities exist in our country," wrote The Leadership Conference on Civil and Human Rights. "For many Americans, the tragedy made visible the unfinished struggle to achieve racial equality and economic justice." With that crisis, suddenly the nation was forced to confront a reality many might not have previously known or were simply in denial.

When it comes to a conversation on race, some of our participants might find themselves saying, "I don't want to be in this conversation on race. Why did I come? I need to get out of here. This conversation is making me feel very vulnerable, raw, and open, and I have no way of sealing the wound." These are some of the ways that the healing crisis makes us feel. So, what's the benefit of going through the crisis?

If we allow ourselves to walk through the discomfort, what we find on the other end is an aware, race-literate and awake human being who will never see the world or this thing we call race in the same way again. What we encounter is someone with a deeper understanding of what it means to be human, a person of color, and American in today's world, and of how this land we share is different for everyone. It opens us to the realization that, while we will never know everything there is to know about race in America, everything we learn makes a difference.

CHAPTER 16
WHEN IT SEEMS ENDLESS

There are times when dealing with race seems endless and hopeless. The problem seems so big that we feel we will drown in it. Don't try to tackle the problem all at once. Indeed, no one person can. But if each of us picks up the mantle, we can make a vast collective difference. Beginning with ourselves, engaging in self-reflection and inspired dialogue, we can help dismantle the wall of separation by removing our personal "brick." If we each take responsibility for doing that, eventually the wall will crumble.

We can then use the old bricks to build a nation-home that is worthy of all of us. We can use our bricks to build a nation in which public safety is about keeping all people safe. We can build good schools and an educational system that works for all children. We can build a healthcare system that is truly accessible to all. And we can build organizations that offer a living wage because all of the above affect the lives and health of people of color.

It takes considerable energy to maintain a dysfunction. When we liberate ourselves, we find the energy to be creative, to find solutions, and to engage in more empowering endeavors. Don't give up. Race consciousness is a process of lifelong learning.

Our five-hundred-year-old racial legacy is not relegated to the past. Indeed, the residue of our racist policies and institutions are still with us today. However, when we understand this past, we can make a difference in the present and can change our collective future.

CHAPTER 17
CREATING A VISION

It is said that without a vision, we perish. Indeed, a vision of what is possible encourages participants to keep the conversation open and creating new possibilities, and it invites us to find our place in the race and health conversation. The purpose of creating a vision is to give the participants an opportunity to imagine what their organization would be like if they could have honest conversations about race — and thereby motivate them to implement conditions that would make it easier to have that conversation. It is also to understand how the new efforts will help the organization serve patients/clients better. The easiest way to create a vision is to imagine the best possible outcome for our organization and the people we serve.

QUESTIONS TO CONSIDER

What needs to happen to improve health in communities of color?

What do we see as possibilities with this topic?

What is missing?

Who is missing from the conversation?

What might our role be in the race and health equity conversation?

It is important that we share our vision, no matter how outlandish. Somewhere between our dream and reality lies a new world of possibilities.

CHAPTER 18
TAKING ACTION

Conversations are just the beginning. Institutions, organizations, and communities need to pool our energies and our resources together to take action — and to take *inspired* action — to change the health of the community. What action will we take? Dreams and visions are great, but actions are essential to change. What participants in this conversation commit to can range from continuing to learn about the nation's history and its impact on health, to becoming more self-reflective. Participants can commito to leading conversations on race and healthcare in their institutions, writing books, holding seminars and a whole host of activities.

One thoughtful participant, a pharmacist said this about her commitment: "After doing a nine-week program on healing from racism with Milagros Phillips, I realized that the only way I could use white privilege in a positive way was to speak out against it. I learned that I had to work to educate white people about systemic racism; otherwise, I was leaving nonwhite people to do it, which is not fair. Now I think more about how my words and actions can either contribute to racism or can help to dismantle it. I think the only way to counter racism or to make race a part of the conversation in my field (healthcare) or society, in general, is to educate people about the effects of racism on all of us and to make it safe to discuss the topic. We have to take the defensiveness and blame out of the equation and acknowledge how racism harms us all in different ways: it causes discrimination against people of color and fragility and infantilism in white people. Then and only then can we talk about how to move forward and create a better and more just society for everyone."

I worked on a project in 2016 where Louisiana's entire health department and the community-based organizations it works with had engaged in antiracism training. Their race literacy was having a tremendous impact on the way these organizations looked at race prompting them to create new action plans to serve their patients/clients. Race literacy can be a powerful way to take action. As testing supervisor Julie Fitch noted:

"The Louisiana Office of Public Health-STD/HIV Program and its partner organizations have been actively engaged in a process to address HIV disparities in our state, particularly as they impact communities of color, since 2013. As part of this effort, Undoing Racism workshops by the People's Institute for Survival and Beyond have been offered to SHP staff and community-based organizations."

There are many ways for an organization to take action. The example above illustrates how health departments around the nation can enhance their race literacy, as a way of becoming more effective in their efforts.

Race Demystified is a program I have offered for the last fifteen years to colleges and universities, community-based organizations, and corporations around the country. The program is customized to fit individual organizations because different organizations have different needs. Race Demystified is a comprehensive two-day intensive experience, and it is also offered as a one-day program. It uses a nonconfrontational approach to race that leaves participants empowered and inspired, regardless of their race.

Speaking race in healthcare means going directly to communities of color and speaking to the community members. It means becoming race literate as a way of being more proficient in our race conversations. It means engaging community members in conversations that include race as a health factor. It means educating clergy to think differently about the health of the members of their religious community. It means addressing the stigma that still exists around various diseases, such as psychiatric conditions and HIV. It requires massive action in the form of a race education campaign that reaches adults and youth. It requires hiring a race expert to support your staff.

It means being proficient in trauma-informed care and addressing intergenerational and historical trauma and sexual-orientation trauma, as non-heterosexuals are often bullied and abused in their communities as well as in their own families. It means having healthcare workers who are not afraid to address and include the impact of race on their patients/clients of color. It requires that healthcare providers receive training in culturally and linguistically appropriate services, diversity, and race. It requires all healthcare workers to treat all patients/clients with respect and to offer them all the information they have available about treatments and medications. It means helping to defuse shame and fear through education, compassion, and care.

It may help to form a community to find new and creative ways to maintain people of color in care. It means hiring experts to help start the conversations. There is a great deal of action that can be taken to turn the tide of healthcare in communities of color. It all begins with a willingness to put race in the conversation.

Everyone can do something right where they are. Everyone has the power to bring about change and compassionately affect the lives of those around them. So, what will we say we did to turn the tide of race and health in our nation? What legacy will we leave behind?

If you would like to schedule a training based on this manual, or any of Milagros' programs, email info@MilagrosPhillips.com. Visit: www.MilagrosPhllips.com to learn more about Milagros' Seminars and programs

BECOMING A LIVING BRIDGE

Each one of us has a wonderful opportunity to become a living bridge to peace and well-being. Our conversations on race are vital to begin that process. A bridge is a connector. It stands in troubled water with unwavering strength, conviction, and stillness. Moreover, a bridge stands between the shadow and the light, facing day and night with the same conviction to see that all who need to cross can do so. And it allows us to explore new lands and new opportunities by being the connecting structure to solid ground.

As living bridges, we create opportunities for people to come together for conversation and sharing. We hold a vision of wholeness for ourselves that allows others to be authentic with us, and we allow ourselves and others the freedom to feel. We believe in people's ability to change, and we trust those changes will take place in their own time. While we may want others to come to the table to speak about race *now*, we know they will do so when they are ready. But this does not keep us from offering them the opportunity to become race literate, because we know it makes a difference.

CHAPTER 19
CONCLUSION

Things have been so unbalanced for so long that, to bring them back to center, we must consider race as part of every decision we make as a nation. As mentioned before in this book, race must be considered in every part of the healthcare conversation. We must consider the impact our actions will have on people at the lowest socioeconomic levels, which most often means people of color. Before embarking on research, we must consider race. When meeting with patients/clients, we must consider race. Before writing another history book, we must consider the impact of telling yet another Eurocentric tale and what that tale would be like if told by people of color. We must consider who is at the table when policies are made, and laws are written. We must consider those who are most vulnerable in our society, who most often are people of color. When looking at the leadership in our organizations, we must consider race. At all points on the health-care continuum, those with the worst health outcomes must be considered as part of the conversation.

Human beings are creatures of community. So when it comes to creating, we create for that which is around us, for that which benefits us, and for those with whom we are involved. This doesn't make us bad people; it simply makes us human. However, when it comes to race, we must be intentional, as those in power are often white and lack the information and experience to lead in this arena.

But human beings are also creatures of imagination, with the capacity to step into someone else's shoes. We have the power of vision, which can expand our reach to other universes. Consider how our healthcare system could change if we made race a leading part of every important conversation and decision. What would happen if we took every component of our society and measured every institution by how it's serving *all* Americans? As a result, we would begin to adjust, change, and transform. Who might we become as people and as a nation? What legacy of health and well-being might we leave our nation?

In conclusion, everyone can do something to make a difference. Together we are unstoppable!

RECOMMENDATIONS

For healthcare institutions to become more effective in including race in the healthcare conversation they will have to be honest about the role of race in the health of their patients/clients. Race will have to take precedence until a more equitable system can exist in our nation. Organizations will have to commit to allowing their members to speak honestly, without repercussions or fear of isolation and job loss. Policies and procedures will need to be scrutinized. It is recommended that organizations hire professionals to help lead the initial conversations on race and train some of their employees to continue those conversations, to ask race-related questions, and to understand how different cultures interact with healthcare.

Long-term organizational commitments will have to be made to invest in race-literacy programs. Organizations will have to ensure that all of their members attend race training programs, without exception. From the board president and founders to donors and employees, all members of the organization will need to engage in educational programs that explore the connection between race and health.

Establish trust by building relationships with the community. It is recommended that organizations develop community forums to inform and educate. Before embarking on another event, ask community members what would be most helpful to them in bringing awareness of the impact of race on their health. Listen and act on what you hear. Go out into the community and establish relationships. Collaborate with local and national organizations. And to share resources and information, establish a community race and health newsletter.

To receive the FREE MANUAL 8 ESSENTIALS TO A RACE CONVERSATION that goes with this book visit:
www.MilagrosPhillips.com
If you would like to schedule a training based on this, or to learn more about Milagros' seminars, and programs

REFERENCES

Note: Most sources listed are under the institutions that issued them regardless of whether they have named authors or editors.

Center for Nonviolent Communication, "Feelings Inventory." 2005.
http://www.cnvc.org/Training/feelings-inventory.

Centers for Disease Control and Prevention, "Fast Facts: HIV Among African-Americans."
https://www.cdc.gov/hiv/group/racialethnic/africanamericans/index.html.

Centers for Disease Control and Prevention, Mathews, T.J., M.S.; MacDorman, Marian F., Ph.D.; "Leading Causes of Infant Death," and Marie E. Thoma, Ph.D., Infant Mortality Statistics From the 2013 Period Linked Birth/Infant Death Data Set Division of Vital Statistics National Vital Statistic Report, Volume 64 Number 9, https://www.cdc.gov/nchs/data/nvsr/nvsr64/nvsr64_09.pdf.

Centers for Disease Control and Prevention, "Reproductive Health: Infant Mortality."
http://www.cdc.gov/reproductivehealth/MaternalInfantHealth/InfantMortality.htm.

Crisis Prevention Institute, Trauma-informed Care Resource Guide. 2017.

Centers for Disease Control and Prevention, HIV Among African-Americans.

https://www.cdc.gov/hiv/group/racialethnic/africaname ricans/index.html

DeGruy, Joy, *Post Traumatic Slave Syndrome: America's Legacy of Enduring Injury and Healing*. Joy DeGruy Publications, 2005.

Department of Health and Human Services, "National Culturally and Linguistically Appropriate Services Standards."
https://www.thinkculturalhealth.hhs.gov/clas/standards.

Elek, Jennifer K., and Paula Hannaford-Agor, "Implicit Bias and the American Juror." *Court Review* 51, no. 3 (2015): 116–121.
http://aja.ncsc.dni.us/publications/courtrv/cr51-3/CR51-3Elek.pdf.

Health Resources and Services Administration, "National HIV/AIDS Strategy: Updated to 2020, HRSA Implementation." 2015. https://hab.hrsa.gov/about-ryan-white-hivaids-program/national-hivaids-strategy-updated-2020.

Institute of Medicine. Brian D. Smedley, Adrienne Y. Stith, and Alan R. Nelson, eds., *Unequal Treatment: Confronting Racial and Ethnic Disparities in Healthcare*. Washington: National Academies Press, 2002.
http://www.nationalacademies.org/hmd/Reports/2002/Unequal-Treatment-Confronting-Racial-and-Ethnic-Disparities-in-Health-Care.aspx.

Leadership Conference on Civil and Human Rights, "Poverty and Hurricane Katrina, Civil Rights Implications of Rebuilding the Gulf Coast."
http://www.civilrights.org/poverty/katrina/.

LGBTQ Nation. Damon L. Jacobs, "Revealing data shows huge racial divide in HIV prevention meds usage." June 21, 2016. http://www.lgbtqnation.com/2016/06/revealing-data-shows-huge-racial-divide-hiv-prevention-meds-usage/.

Pew Research Center. Eilene Patten, "The black-white and urban-rural divides in perceptions of racial fairness," *FactTank News in the Numbers*, August 28, 2013.

http://www.pewresearch.org/fact-tank/2013/08/28/the-black-white-and-urban-rural-divides-in-perceptions-of-racial-fairness/.

Pew Research Center, "On Views of Race and Inequality, Blacks and Whites Are Worlds Apart." Pew Research Center Social & Demographic Trends, June 21, 2016. http://www.pewsocialtrends.org/2016/06/27/on-views-of-race-and-inequality-blacks-and-whites-are-worlds-apart/.

Phillips, Milagros, *Eight Stages to Healing Race in America*.

Skloot, Rebecca, *The Immortal Life of Henrietta Lacks*. New York: Crown Publishers, 2010.

Teen Vogue. Lincoln Anthony Blades, "Trauma From Slavery Can Actually Be Passed Down Through Your Genes: You can get PTSD from your ancestors." May 31,

2016. http://www.teenvogue.com/story/slavery-trauma-inherited-genetics.

UNAIDS, "Mayors from Around the World Sign Paris Declaration to End AIDS/HIV." Press release, December 1, 2014. http://www.unaids.org/en/resources/presscentre/pressreleaseandstatementarchive/2014/december/20141201_PR_citiesreport.

Harvard Health Publishing, Harvard Medical School, Havard Men's Health Watch "Breath Meditation: A great way to relieve stress. April 2014. https://www.health.harvard.edu/mind-and-mood/breath-meditation-a-great-way-to-relieve-stress

W. M. Byrd and L. A Clayton, "Race, medicine, and healthcare in the United States: a historical survey."

Journal of the National Medical Association, 2001. https://www.ncbi.nlm.nih.gov/pmc/articles/PMC2593958/

Unnatural Causes: Is Inequality Making Us Sick, episode 2, "When the Bough Breaks." California News Reel, 2008. http://newsreel.org/video/UNNATURAL-CAUSES.

Washington, Harriet A., Medical Apartheid: The Dark History of Medical Experimentation on Black Americans from Colonial Times to the Present. New York: Doubleday,2006.

WebMD. Daniel J. DeNoon, "Why 7 Deadly Diseases Strike Blacks Most." Published Feb. 7, 2005. http://www.webmd.com/hypertension-high-blood-pressure/features/why-7-deadly-diseases-strike-blacks-most.

Wikipedia, "List of Countries by Infant Mortality Rate." Last accessed DATE. https://en.wikipedia.org/wiki/List_of_countries_by_infant_mortality_rate.

World Health Organization, "World Health Statistics 2016 data visualization dashboard." Last accessed DATE. http://apps.who.int/gho/data/node.sdg.3-2-viz?lang=en.

Kathryn Doyle, Racially biased cancer doctors spend less time with black patients." Health News, June 24, 2016. https://www.reuters.com/article/us-health-racialbias-cancer/racially-biased-cancer-doctors-spend-less-time-with-black-patients-idUSKCN0ZA3N9

Dictionary references

RACE, https://www.merriam-webster.com/dictionary/race

RACISM, https://www.merriam-webster.com/dictionary/racism

RACIST, https://en.oxforddictionaries.com/definition/racist

PREJUDICE, https://en.oxforddictionaries.com/definition/prejudice

BIAS, https://en.oxforddictionaries.com/definition/bias

IMPLICIT BIAS, "Understanding Implicit Bias." https://kirwaninstitute.osu.edu/research/understanding-implicit-bias/

EXPLICIT BIAS, Perceptions Institute. https://perception.org/research/explicit-bias/

http://www.ncsc.org/~/media/Files/PDF/Topics/Gender%20and%20Racial%20Fairness/Implicit%20Bias%20FAQs%20rev.ashx

DISCRIMINATION, https://en.oxforddictionaries.com/definition/discrimination

WHITE PRIVILEGE, https://en.wikipedia.org/wiki/White_privilege

ABOUT THE AUTHOR

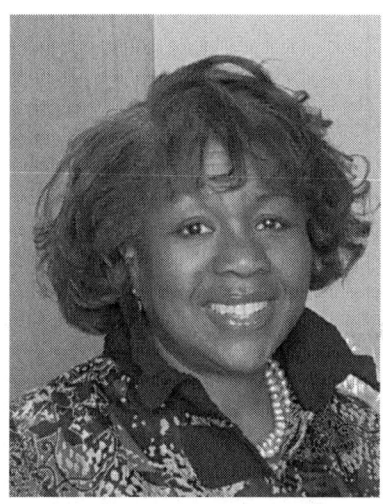

Milagros Phillips is the author of *Eleven Reasons to Become Race Literate: A Pocket Guide to a New Conversation* and *Eight Essentials to a Race Conversation: A Manual to a New Dialogue*. She is a Diversity & Race Coach and has spent the last twenty-five years bringing race literacy to colleges, universities, national leaders, corporations, and nonprofit organizations with her historically grounded, race-based seminars and programs. A speaker, an artist, and a freelance consultant, she may be reached at **info@milagrosphillips.com www.MilagrosPhillips.com. Milagros is also a TEDx speaker.**

A Manual for a New Dialogue

Made in the USA
Middletown, DE
15 June 2020